Eating Not Eating

By David Kenneth
&
Kimberly Swinson

Introduction

Eating Not Eating offers a comprehensive fasting guide to help you achieve your fasting goals, inner-stand the ins-and-outs of fasting, and provide you with valuable tips and tricks to make the process as easy and successful as possible. With Eating Not Eating, you can fast with confidence and get the most out of your fasting journey. This guide will help you detox and prepare to live a happy, joyful, free life, full of life! Eating Not Eating is a road map for intuitive self healers to guide themselves into success and to discover their greatest gift, their bodies natural healing capabilities through fasting and enema cleanses. When we cleanse our Body Temple from all the processed toxic foods, we prepare it for a complete awakening. We can turn our dis-ease into ease when we commit to loving ourselves in such a way that we only put what is for our highest good into our Body Temple.

Eating and Fasting Journal

An eating journal is a good way to keep track of what you eat and how it makes you feel. Get to know yourself and how eating and fasting treats your Body Temple. Learning how each item you eat has its effect on your energy, feelings and mood. Write down in your journal everything you eat, and when you eat it. Keep track of how you feel after eating and the next day. Journaling about your bowel movements schedule and consistency. Write out your fasting commitments and your experience. Having this information down helps one to go back and see with their own experience. We recommend you do your own research, but we will provide you with a foundation. We all have access to looking up whatever we want. Learn about all foods you are eating and what effect they have on your Temple. If you don't know what an ingredient is, put it into Google and search its side effects. Or tune into your inner guidance and ask yourself if it is for your highest good. What we choose to put into our Body Temple effects ALL aspects of us as the physical and spiritual bodies are inherently connected.

Live Life Happy, Blissful, Healthy and Free!!!!!!!

Eating

Putting food in the mouth, chewing and swallowing it. Chew until the food is broken down into liquid. This requires eating and chewing mindfully, not distracted by our phones, etc. We eat to feed our Body Temple, which is our church, house and vehicle. We only get one in this lifetime. Practice treating it well and doing no harm. It is your choice what you feed yourself. What we choose to eat either contributes to our Body Temple being at ease or in dis-ease. Practice not eating to fullness. Practice eating only two meals a day. Practice only eating when you are hungry

What to Eat

Consume only foods that are good for the Body Temple.

Raw organic simple ingredients are the best.

Raw fruit and vegetables that contain the seeds are live food and give life to us.

If something is seedless, it has been genetically modified and is not for the Body Temple's highest good.

Organic raw seeds and nuts

Raw seaweed
Superfood powders
Raw organic nut butters
Sprouted grains
Cold-pressed oils and juices
Foods that cause the body to be
alkaline
Eat local organic produce as much
as possible within a hundred mile
range
Change your lifestyle a little each
day to eat more healthily

Benefits of an Alkaline Diet:
1. Improved Bone Health
2. Reduced Risk of Cardiovascular Diseases
3. Management and Elimination of Chronic Disease
4. Huge Increase in Energy Levels
5. Better Digestion
6. Easier Fat Loss
7. Less Pain from Inflammation Related Conditions (like arthritis)
8. Better Moods
9. Slows Down the Degeneration of Cells
10. Prevents Clots and Blockages in the Blood
PLUS! A longer, healthier and more active life!

ALKALINE FRUITS:

Avocado
Grapefruit
Watermelon (with seeds)
Apple (with seeds)
Mango
Bananas (small or burros)
Oranges (Seville with seeds)
Pineapple
Blueberry
Raspberries
Strawberries
Grapes (with seeds)
Cantaloupe (with seeds)
Dragon Fruit
Pomegranate
Kiwi
Pears
Apricots

Cherries
Dates
Papaya
Coconut
Tangerine
Melons (with seeds)
Figs
Lime (key limes preferred)
Lemons (with seeds)
Soursop
Tamarind
Prickly Pear
This is not a comprehensive list.
There may be other alkaline fruits
in your local area as well.
Research or preferrably ask your
inner guidance.
You are your best teacher-learn to
trust yourself.

ALKALINE VEGETABLES ROOTS & GRASSES:

Kale

Arugula

Spinach

Broccoli

Collard Greens

Dandelion Greens

Lettuce (no iceberg)

Zucchini

Yellow Squash

Mushrooms (no shitake)

Cucumbers

Tomatoes-Cherry and Plum

Bell Peppers

Green Onions

Celery

Chlorella and Spirulina

Radishes

Beets

Sprouts

Cilantro

Parsley

Basil

Mint

Thyme

Watercress

Ginger

Sea Moss

Again, this is not a comprehensive list, but a guide

Learn to tune into your own inner guidance to receive answers

NUTS AND SEEDS
Almonds (soaked and husk
removed)
Coconut
Flax Seeds
Chia Seeds
Hemp Seeds
Pumpkin Seeds
Sesame Seeds
Sunflower Seeds
Walnuts
Pecans
Macadamia
Brazil

These are the nuts we like to
consume regularly on the alkaline
diet along with their health benefits:

Macadamia nuts are so healthy
and alkaline.

They are an incredible source of essential fatty acids including Omega 3's and 6's, so a perfect choice for alkaline dieting. They are also alkaline-forming when digested, and provide good amounts of dietary fiber.

Although they are high in fat, macadamia nuts contain primarily monounsaturated fat, which is the heart-healthy type of fat that can help reduce your risk of heart disease and type 2 diabetes.

Macadamia nuts have the highest fat content, making them the most calorific nut and therefore are a great source of energy, and brain power.

A cup or 132g of macadamia nuts contains:

Calories: 945

Protein: 10.3 g

Fat: 100 g
Carbs: 16.9 g
Fiber: 10.6 g
Sugar: 5.46 g
Calcium: 92.4 milligrams (mg)
Iron: 3.5 mg
Magnesium: 156 mg

Walnuts are another alkaline nut to incorporate into an alkaline diet whenever you can. They provide essential fatty acids in addition to protein, fibre, vitamins and minerals.

Plus they are the best nut-source of omega 3, making them one of the more alkaline nuts. Walnuts are also an excellent source of alpha-linolenic acid, the plant-based omega-3 fatty acid.

One ounce of walnuts provides a significant amount of total fat, including monounsaturated and polyunsaturated fats.

A 1-ounce (30-gram) serving of walnuts — about 14 halves — provides the following essential nutrients:

Calories: 185

Water: 4%

Protein: 4.3 grams

Carbs: 3.9 grams

Sugar: 0.7 grams

Fiber: 1.9 grams

Fat: 18.5 grams

Almonds are alkaline forming when digested (we recommend always soaking and sprouting almonds and removing the husk for easier digestion) and provide good amounts of fats, protein, dietary fibre and vitamins & minerals.

Almonds are a fantastic source of antioxidants, magnesium, vitamin E and manganese, plus the fats omega 6, 9, 3 and small amount of saturated fat (80% monounsaturated, 15% polyunsaturated, and 5% saturated)

They are also incredibly high in antioxidants, which help protect cells from oxidative stress, which can damage molecules and contribute to inflammation, aging, and diseases like cancer.

A 1-ounce (28-gram) serving of almonds contains:

Fiber: 3.5 grams

Protein: 6 grams

Fat: 14 grams (9 of which are monounsaturated)

Vitamin E: 37% of the RDI

Manganese: 32% of the RDI

Magnesium: 20% of the RDI
They also contain a decent amount of copper,
vitamin B2 (riboflavin) and phosphorus.

Brazil nuts are an excellent source of nutrition, providing fats, antioxidants, vitamins, and minerals.
They're particularly high in selenium, a mineral with potent antioxidant properties. Eating Brazil nuts may reduce inflammation, support brain function, and improve your thyroid function and heart health .
Brazil nuts provide good amounts of fats in addition to protein, fiber, vitamins and minerals.
They are an alkaline nut that contains the highest amount of

selenium than any other nut, with a single nut containing almost 200% of your daily needs.

Selenium is a powerful antioxidant that helps protect cells from oxidative damage, supports the immune system and may reduce the risk of certain cancers. Plus it also helps with thyroid health and metabolism.

These are one of my favorites because you don't need to eat a lot to get that selenium hit!

A 1-ounce (28-gram) serving of Brazil nuts contains the following nutrients:

Calories: 187
Protein: 4.1 grams
Fat: 19 gram
Carbs: 3.3 grams
Fiber: 2.1 grams
Selenium: 989% daily value (DV)

Copper: 55% DV
Magnesium: 25% DV
Phosphorus: 16% DV
Manganese: 15% DV
Zinc: 10% DV
Thiamine: 15% DV
Vitamin E: 11% DV

Pecan Nuts
Pecans are rich in antioxidants, which can help delay the progression of degenerative neurological diseases like Amyotrophic Lateral Sclerosis (ALS), also known as Lou Gehrig's disease. Pecans can also help lower LDL levels.
Pecans are packed with vitamins and minerals like Vitamin E, manganese, magnesium, phosphorus, zinc, iron, and calcium. All these nutrients can

help boost your immunity and keep you healthy. Pecans have also been found to contain high levels of dietary fiber which is beneficial for your digestive health as it removes toxins from our bodies. Additionally, studies have found that consumption of pecans has been linked to reduced risk of certain cancers and heart disease. They can also help lower cholesterol levels, which helps reduce your risk of stroke and other cardiovascular problems. Furthermore, they are a great source of healthy fats that can help keep your skin looking youthful.

One ounce (28 grams) of pecans contains the following nutritional value:

Calories: 196

Protein: 2.5 grams

Fat: 20.5 grams
Carbs: 4 grams
Fiber: 2.7 grams
Copper: 38% of the Daily Value (DV)
Thiamine (vitamin B1): 16% of the DV
Zinc: 12% of the DV
Magnesium: 8% of the DV
Phosphorus: 6% of the DV
Iron: 4% of the DV

We have used other nuts as well, but strive not to use Cashews because the outer shells are very acidic and harm those who husk them, which is mainly women and children in India.
We encourage you to research this and make up your own mind as to whether or not you choose to consume them.

OILS

Cold-pressed organic olive oil

Cold-pressed organic coconut oil

Cold-pressed organic avocado oil

List in your Journal what you like to
eat that you know is good for you

What Not to Eat

Foods that cause the body to be acidic

Practice avoiding fast food, processed food, breads, refined sugars, artificial coloring and flavors, fried, soda, canned foods, alcohol, anything pasteurized, coffee, hot drinks and preservatives, nutritional yeast and most things that are man made. 'Natural flavorings' can be many different things, including MSG…don't trust them.

Milk and its products can cause mucus and inflammation, as it is pasteurized and heavily processed.

Heated oil is not good for the Body Temple .

Eating dead rotting animal flesh will cause suffering .

If the ingredient is unknown search it up and its side effects.
Don't mix too many foods together, keep it simple for your digestion.
Do not eat foods that have to be shipped in from far away countries.

ACIDIC FOODS & OTHER HARMFUL COOKING HABITS TO AVOID

Fried Foods

All food prepared on an outdoor grill or open fire (you are exposed to two main carcinogens: heterocyclic aromatic hydrocarbons (HCAs) and polycyclic aromatic hydrocarbons (PAHs) Studies show HCAs and PAHs cause changes in the DNA that may increase the risk of cancer.

ALL Meat

Poultry

Sugar
Gluten
Margarine
All Seed Oils
Fish & Seafood
Eggs
ALL Dairy Products
Grains (especially wheat)
Alcohol, Wine and Beer
ALL Soda Pop, (They contain harmful sugars, dyes and carbonation that is harmful for the Body Temple)
Coffee
ALL Sugar Drinks
ALL Energy Drinks
ALL Carbonated Drinks
ALL Artificial Sweeteners like Equal, Sweet & Low, Nutra Sweet, etc.
Pastries
Vinegar

ALL Canned Foods
ALL Corn and Corn Products
including Corn Syrup
ALL breads are toxic unless grains
are sprouted and the sprouted
grains are dehydrated or baked in
the sun
Nutritional Yeast
All Processed Foods
Peanuts and Peanut Butter

Here are reasons we encourage
everyone to avoid peanuts.
They are incredibly vulnerable to
mold, during the growing,
harvesting and storage phases,
and over 25 strains of bacteria are
commonly found on them.
One particular mold, a carcinogen
called aflatoxin, a natural toxin
produced by certain strains of the
mold, is very concerning.

These acid-forming molds have no place in an alkaline diet (where mold is one thing we are definitely trying to avoid!).

Not only is aflatoxin consumption linked to cancer, but it can also stunt the growth of children and cause liver toxicity.

It is especially dangerous for pregnant women, as aflatoxin has been linked to stillbirths and low birth weights. It can also cause skin rashes, pale skin, hair loss, and abdominal pain in adults.

And when you think about how peanuts are most often consumed – as peanut butter (highly concentrated acidic peanuts!), it's never a good choice.

Even if you purchase organic peanuts or peanut butter, it is still highly acidic and not a wise choice

to consume if you want to have a healthy Body Temple.
What these manufacturers fail to mention is that they use the peanuts with less mold for your cocktail peanuts, and the ones with more mold for peanut butter- since it gets mashed up anyway!
The problem is that the mold spores in the peanuts, while they may not be visible to the naked eye, are still present.
As you eat them, these microscopic organisms release their toxins into your system which can cause a myriad of health problems.

A good rule of thumb we strive to always follow...if nature didn't make it, we don't take it!

List in your Journal what you eat
that is not good for your Body
Temple

Cancer
It grows, feeds and thrives off of an
Acidic Body Temple
It cannot survive and disappears
with a Alkaline Body Temple
Best to eat foods that promote an
Alkaline Body Temple
Cancer and other autoimmune
diseases can be avoided and cured
with fasting and eating properly

Cravings
What you desire to eat may not be
your desires
It may be a habit or tradition
It could be the worms and
parasites requests for what they
like
Practice avoiding your cravings,
work on replacing them with food
that is good for you
Write a list in your Journal of your
Cravings.
Ask yourself WHY you are craving
these foods and see what answers
come when you journal.

Fasting

The practice of abstaining from the consumption of all or some types of food.

Types of Fasting

Water Fast - Only Drinking Water

Liquid Fast - Only Drinking Liquids

Dry Fast - No Food, No Liquid (including water)

Mono Fasting - Eating only one kind of food

Karma Fasting - Not eating foods that cause you harm or caused harm of another.

Intermittent Fasting - Prolonging the time between eating, eating only for a short period during the day (1-8 hrs) and fasting the rest.

Multiple Day Fast - Fasting many days - 3 Day Fast, 5 Day fast, 7 Day Fast - 40 Day Fast

Forever Fast - Breatharianism

Fasting Benefits
Improved Heath
Increased Energy
Cures Disease and Ailments
Boosts Weight Loss
Enhances Brain Function
Reduces Inflammation
Improves Digestion
Reduces Blood Pressure
Improves Insulin Sensitivity
Triggers Autophagy
Slows Aging Process
Increase Human Growth Hormone

When one stops eating, the energy going to digestion stops and the body switches over to healing.

Then the body starts to heal the problem spots like inflammation, tumors and cancer.

Consult a physician if you have any of these conditions before attempting a multiple day fast:
Insulin dependent
Hypoglycemic
On menstrual cycle (From my experience fasting on my cycle was not harmful, it just zapped my energy, listen to your own inner guidance)
Taking medications

Tips for Fasting/Breaking Fast
Use filtered spring water with
minerals if possible
Panakos deep seawater is a good
supplement as it contains
electrolytes and minerals.
Break fast with organic raw juice or
organic fresh fruit and slowly ease
into eating.

Practice

Life is a series of practices

Each day is a new day for

practicing

Remember to be gentle on self

Judging ourselves harshly does not

help in this process

Treat yourself with compassion and

kindness

If you feel the need to eat and

cannot go through with the fast, eat

and practice another day

Having a clear intention and
making a commitment to yourself
With water fast, drinking water
when feeling hungry can help
during fasting time
Returning to our intention mindfully
focuses our attention to the reason
we chose to fast
Are you ready to love your Body
Temple and yourself more?
Are you willing to do what it takes
to detox your Body Temple from all
the harmful processed foods and
chemicals?

Intermittent Fasting
Separating the eating and not
eating times.
While asleep one does not eat or
drink this is the Sleeping Fast.
Breakfast is the breaking of the
sleeping fast.
Practice not breaking your fast with
breakfast because breakfast is
break fast.
Practice Eating Brunch =
Breakfast/Lunch
First meal around 10am.
Practice Eating Linner =
Lunch/Dinner.
Last meal around 3pm
OR
Practice first meal around noon,
and last meal around 5pm

These are just ideas, tune into
YOUR inner guidance and Body
Temple wisdom
Play around with the times to what
is in the flow of life
The fast starts after finished eating
for the day
The goal would be to shorten the
time one eats and lengthen the
time one is not eating
Eating all needed within the eating
time period
Shortening the eating time, practice
eight, six, four or two hours
Lengthening the fasting time twenty
or twenty-two hours

The fasting time can be done dry,
or with water
Returning to your intention helps
the will power
Journal your progress each day
The fasting time can be done dry,
liquid or just water
Returning to your intention helps
the will power
The body starts burning sugars
stabilizing blood sugar levels
The intestines switch from digest to
repair.

One Day Fast
24 hours of Fasting
Energy is up and so is mood and
cognitive functions
Fat burning kicks in and the liver
makes ketones
New brain cells are created
Lengthening your Intermittent
fasting to a whole day fast.

Multiple Day Fast
After doing a 24 hour fast next practice for two days, then try three or if you are ready jump to a five day fast and work your way up to the 7 day fast.
48 hours Insulin sensitivity super boost, less inflammation, atrophy healing and protein sparing, killing cancer cells.

Day Two Fast Benefits
Increase in Brain-derived neurotrophic factor (BDNF) plays an important role in neuronal survival and growth, serves as a neurotransmitter modulator, and participates in neuronal plasticity, which is essential for learning and memory.

Human growth hormone (HGH) is a natural hormone your pituitary gland releases that promotes growth in children, helps maintain normal body structure in adults and plays a role in metabolism in both children and adults.

Increase in Autophagy (Real clean up starts to occur. Break down TAu proteins, amyloid, alpha synucleins, and prime glial cells.

Helps with PTSD, Parkinson's, Alzheimer's,Concusions, Lewy body dementia, etc. breaks down aggregates in the brain and clears them out)

Mitophagy occurs (gets rid of inefficient mitochondria in our cells. Mitochondria produces energy ATP and you want mitochondria to be efficient and produce the number of ATP's it is suppose to. It will start to get rid of things that are damaged and get them out of our system)

Insulin resistance will come down. People who are pre-diabetic/diabetic and insulin resistant will start to improve.

Decrease in fatty liver because you are using fat for fuel and part of that fat will come from the liver and will clear fatty liver if it is not too far advanced

90-95% of energy will come from ketones instead of glucose

Hunger will decrease

Day Three Fast Benefit
Continued increase in autophagy

Reversal of chronic disease

Immune function will reset and improvement of white blood cells and stem cells will help you heal.

The goal of a three day fast is Metabolic Flexibility or a Metabolic Switch. This is the ability for the body to use both glucose and ketones whenever it wants. If you are someone who eats every day you are using insulin most of the time. The purpose of a fase is to even out the blood sugar throughout the day. When you stabilize the blood sugar the body becomes hybrid, using ketones as fuel. The body becomes like a hybrid versus just using gas (food) as fuel.

Clean the brain and reset energy
Improves Immune system
Repairs damaged cells
Removes dysfunctional cells and pathogens
Reduces (neuro) inflammation
Increase autophagy (breaks down cells and pathogens)
Decrease auto-immune disease
Benefits gut flora
Increases DNA repair

After 72 hours of fasting the Immune system regenerates as does the brain, creating new stem cells

Journal your experience and thoughts during your fasts. Look at these commitments like a sacred ceremony, because it is! You are committing to honoring the sacred gift of life and treating your Body Temple with respect and honor. You are committing to listening to your sacred Body Temple. To treat each day like a sacred ceremony with what you choose to gift (eat and drink) to your Body Temple, remembering you are a unique emanation of Source Creator. Ask your Body Temple what it needs. Tune into it. This sacred gift of life is a blessing! When you love your Body Temple you are loving God. Love yourself with all your heart, mind, and strength. Honor life by honoring your Body Temple.

7 Day Fast

A seven day water fast and enema cleanse will help remove the guck in your Body Temple and prepare your body for a Raw Food dis-ease free life.

This is a BIG step. It will require a lot of self discipline. We recommend not attempting this step if you have not practiced intermittent and/or shorter fasts first. It is best to do this seven day complete detox and cleanse when you have a space all to yourself where no one else is eating or preparing food around you for the duration of the fast and no major commitments like work.

This kind of fast will help remove parasites and worms from the body.

Removing the internal cravings for fried salty, sugary foods and processed foods and harmful addictive chemicals.

Along with two enemas each day to cleanse the colon and ten to fifteen minutes nude sunbathing (front and back) each day for optimal results.

This is a complete reset for the Body Temple if done properly.

We recommend purchasing spring water or finding a natural spring to fill large water containers to do your seven day fast. Spring water contains necessary minerals that the body needs to stay energized and healthy during the fasting period. Tap water is often treated with chlorine, fluoride and sometimes other chemicals as well so it is advised to not ever use this water to drink unless you have a really good filtering system at home that removes these.

A water fast means ONLY water. No honey, tea, coffee, oils or anything else during this seven day fast. Drink room temperature spring or VERY good filtered water that still contains minerals as needed.

You will need to purchase an at home enema kit. We like the kits that have a bag you can fill with water as they are easier to take when traveling. You can typically find one for around $30 online. We do not recommend coffee enemas. From my experience, doing a coffee enema is like drinking a cup of coffee. After doing it one time I felt jittery and had a difficult time sleeping. Coffee is also one of the most heavily pesticide sprayed crops, so best to stay away from chemicals when doing a cleanse.

Read enema bag instructions prior to attempting this step. Use two cups of spring water heated to body temperature, around 98-100* F or 37-38* C. DO NOT USE HOT

WATER. You can warm the water in the sun if done during the summer for added charging benefits. Add two teaspoons of sea salt to the water and mix well. Pour into enema bag, making sure the clamp is closed tightly. Hang the enema bag on a nail or hook or have someone hold it about 12 to 18 inches above your rectum. Insert the enema nozzle into rectum (you can use coconut oil or other oil to lube. I like coconut oil) Insert the end of the hose into rectum. Release the water stopper on the enema hose while on all fours. I like to stick my butt in the air like a stink bug.

Relax as best you can and allow all the water to flow into your body. DEEP BREATHS! Stay in this position for at least 15 minutes. When time is up, go ahead and release the water and toxins on the toilet. You might be here for a bit, so get comfy! Do one in the morning and one in the evening each day of the fast. You want the water of your enema to be CLEAR on day seven. If it is not, consider continuing to fast with enemas until it is. This is the complete detox. This is what will rid your Body Temple of parasites and completely cleanse it to prepare it for transitioning to eating True Raw.

During this process treat it like you
would a ceremony.
Set your intention.
Create a sacred space and have all
the items ready for you to dive in
and heal yourself fully.

Items needed and recommended:
1. A journal and pen
2. Enough spring water to drink and do two enemas (two cups of water per enema) each day
3. A medium pot to be able to heat water in (not aluminum or anything non stick as these contain harmful chemicals) on a hot plate, stove or preferably in the sun
4. An Enema Kit
5. Sea or Himalayan Salt (Do not use iodized table salt)
6. Sage and lighter to clear the energy in your space each day
7. Any crystals or totems that will help you remember this is a sacred ceremony
8. An area set aside to create an alter

Day Fast
A 40 day juice fast will help prepare
your body for a raw eating life
This helps remove the guck stuck
from eating cooked foods
I have not done this fast yet so I
will not talk about it here in detail
until I do my research

Forever Fast - Breatharianism
Not Eating
Not Drinking
Receiving the Nectar
from the Environment

This Practice takes a lot of practice
and preparation

From Eating Everything to Eating
Nothing
Through the path of Vegetarian
To Vegan
To True Raw
To Fruitarian
To Liquidarian
To Breatharian

Remember: Life is the Ceremony
and YOU are the Medicine!

Remember you are not alone.

We are here for you.

We have fasting retreats and
programs on our website
Thesdic.org

David and Kimberly
Have spent a lifetime learning

They came here to share that
wisdom picked up along the way.

Creating a Loves School
And
Loves Services
On
The Sdic Inc
Webpage for all to enjoy
TheSdic.org

They also have more books
available there.